Don't Panic!

5 Things Every Birth Partner Needs to Know

by
Rena Gough

Great thanks go to my husband, Andy, for supporting me in all my crazy dreams, looking after our 3 bundles of joy (can you still call them that if they are 8, 6 and 4?!) while I worked on my writing, and for just being my biggest fan.

One day I hope my kids will read this book, and they will be proud of the difference it has made to the birth of so many babies. I have written it so my son feels confident he has got what it takes to be the birth partner she needs him to be, and so my daughters will grow up trusting in birth – should they choose to have children, obviously!

---

with special thanks to
Saveria: **www.saveria.uk**
for her invaluable proofreading skills

Visit **www.keepcalmandbirthon.com** for more books including

The Pregnancy Book: 8 Tips for a Happy Pregnancy

Keep Calm and Birth On: 10 Ways to Survive Giving Birth

CONTENTS

INTRODUCTION

Congratulations! Being asked to be a birth partner is a great privilege which comes with great responsibility. Yep, being a birth partner is more than getting your hand squeezed and randomly shouting 'Push!!!' at the end. You are a key part of the birth and your support will be invaluable to the lady concerned, as long as you know what to do and when. Whether you are the dad, the grandparent, the aunty, the not-really-related aunty or the adoptive parents, it doesn't matter, this book will give you a detailed insight into what she will go through, what she needs from you, ways you can support her emotionally and physically, and how you can help her bring this baby into the world with as little drama as possible.

Don't worry, it is actually an easier job than it sounds. You just need to read this book. It will give you a good understanding of how the female body gives birth, what makes it work better and what makes it shut down, and it will explain how to create a good environment around the birthing lady, how to make sure she gets everything she needs and how to step up as her advocate if she needs you to. Because that it is all you need to know and know how to do, really.

It should only take you around half an hour to read this book. It is not deep or intense, and it is not meant to confuse you with a million different scenarios and possible outcomes. It is here to give you the confidence your pregnant person needs you to have so she can give birth the way she wants.

If she hasn't done so already, reading Keep Calm and Birth On: 10 Ways to Survive Giving Birth will give the pregnant lady in your life an amazing insight into her body and how it will give birth, and arm her with an amazing set of tools to cope with the whole thing.

To make things easier whilst explaining this stuff, I am going to call this pregnant lady Penelope.

So let's go...

WHAT TO DO WHEN LABOUR BEGINS

In the movies and on TV, a woman's waters break all over the floor and then all of a sudden she is in full-blown labour. In real life, this is not how it tends to work. In fact some women's waters don't break at all and their babies are born 'en caul', that is, still in the amniotic sac. What is more likely to happen is that Penelope will get a few uncomfortable twinges, maybe two or three an hour for a while, and at some point she will realise that these are contractions. Early labour is usually nothing like in the movies: it tends to be slow, so it can be quite boring, and really your job at this stage is to make Penelope as comfortable as possible and help her to conserve her energy for later on. Provide plenty of water and light snacks, and let her get on with breathing through each contraction as it happens. If she doesn't realise until they are getting quite intense, this is okay and there is no need to panic or rush, just make her as comfortable as you can as quickly as you can.

The main thing you need to remember is that it is much easier for Penelope to give birth if she is relaxed. That doesn't mean lying on the couch with a brew watching 'Love Island'; it means being in a space and environment that allows her to shut off her mind and relax all the muscles in her body, particularly those in her uterus and around her pelvis. The uterus is a set of muscles. They work exactly like any other muscles in your body, and just like any other muscles in your body, if she can let them work properly then it shouldn't hurt. Take your arm, for example. If you extend your arm, you will notice that the tricep muscle is contracted and the bicep muscle is relaxed. In order to bend your arm you need to relax the tricep muscle and contract the bicep muscle. Easy, no? The two work together smoothly and we go around using our arms all day with no aches and pains. The uterus works in the same way. If you can imagine it as an inflated balloon, there are long muscles that go from the top to the bottom, and circular muscles that go all the way around, concentrated at the bottom to make up the cervix. When Penelope goes into labour, those long muscles are the ones that contract (hence contractions) and those circular muscles need to be relaxed so that they can easily be pulled out of the way of the baby's head, i.e. thin and dilate. The cervix is about 2–3cm long, thick and hard during pregnancy, in order to keep the baby in. When it is time for baby to be born, all of that has to move out of the way. Each contraction is doing a job: it may be trying to shift the baby into the optimum position, it might be causing the cervix to soften, it could be thinning the cervix or it could be dilating. It is important to remember this as many women believe that contractions are only there to dilate their cervix, and therefore if they have been in labour for some time but are not very far dilated, they begin to feel that their body is not working correctly. This is not the case, as those contractions may have had other positive effects that are needed to birth the baby but are not necessarily obvious. It can be important in these circumstances to reassure Penelope that her body is doing exactly what it needs to. Once the cervix has moved out of the way, the baby begins to make its way down the birth canal, ready to be born. We will go over this bit in Chapter 5.

Labour can become extremely painful because, in most cases, women fight the movement of these muscles by tensing. To illustrate this, try the following: bite your back teeth together as hard as you can; you are probably feeling the whole inside of your body tense, in particular your pelvic area. Now extend your arm as you did earlier and this time try to bend it whilst tensing both muscles at the same time. It suddenly becomes a much more difficult task, and your arm probably feels like it is doing a much harder and a much greater job. As well as this, if you spent half an hour using your arm in this way, it would soon be exhausted and achy. If you had no choice but to keep using it in this way, it wouldn't be long before it hurt so much you would want to give in. So you can imagine that if Penelope is tense during a contraction, she will cause those uterine circular muscles to tighten, creating that same resistance as you produced when you tried to bend your arm whilst tensing both muscles. The long muscles can't move the circular muscles effectively, and both sets of muscles become tired and overworked much faster than they would if they were able to work smoothly. It also means that they have to try again to do the job, adding contractions to the labour, i.e. making the labour longer than necessary. Conversely, if Penelope is able to stay relaxed during each contraction and allow the muscles to work together, her labour is likely to be shorter, much less painful and a much more positive experience for both her and the baby (and you!). This is not to say that birth won't take any effort – that would be like asserting that Mo Farah doesn't need to put in any effort when he runs a marathon! – but if Penelope is able to stay as relaxed as possible, then she will find it much easier to cope with each contraction, and her uterus shouldn't get worn out too quickly.

Your job as the birth partner is to facilitate this as much as possible, so Penelope doesn't have to. From where you are to the things going on around you, you need to create the best environment possible for her to relax in. Whilst at home this can be easy to do, using soft lighting and relaxing music, asking people to sit in different rooms when they don't need to be in the same room as her, and generally keeping it peaceful around Penelope. Answer the door and send people away, turn off all the phones, make sure you know where everything you need for the birth is, let the hospital know she is in labour, pack the last-minute things, and tell her how amazing she is and how excited you are. Find yourself something to do but be easily available if she needs you, and very importantly, don't ask her a million questions or expect her to discuss current politics with you! Instead, see if she fancies watching a funny film with you or read a book or magazine. Also remember that she may want to be by herself, and be accepting of the fact that she is likely to keep changing her mind – *about everything*. One minute she will want you on the bed next to her, the next she might tell you to go away. One minute she might be freezing and the next she might be stripping off like there's a heat wave. One minute she will be downing pints of water and the next she will feel sick at the sight of it. *Your job is to not get annoyed*. Even if you think she is acting like the queen of divas, right now she just needs you to say 'Yes, ma'am' and do whatever it is she needs.

Another of your jobs is to keep your eye on the amount of time in between the contractions. You don't need a fancy app for this, just a clock or a watch will do. Start timing them when you think they are getting quite close together. To do this, notice the time when Penelope begins to breathe through a contraction; (there is an explanation of this in Chapter 2 so you know what to look out for), and then notice the time when she begins to breathe through the next one. Do this without asking her to tell you when it starts so you don't disturb her. If it is a gap of 5 minutes or less, then it is probably time to start thinking about calling the midwife if she is birthing at home, or getting ready to go to the birth centre or hospital. They say that for a first-time mum, she should be having roughly three contractions in 10 minutes, so that is a gap of about 3 and a half minutes between the start of each one. They should also be lasting roughly a minute, so once you feel they are getting close enough together, time how long one lasts for. You only need to time the contractions for a short while, half an hour maximum. Don't get too hung up about the numbers and the timings. Instead, listen to her and the noises she makes as labour progresses. If it sounds like things are getting tough, then it is time to call the midwife or the birth centre/hospital.

If she has chosen to birth at home, the relaxing environment can be carried on throughout the labour easily. If she has chosen to go to a birth-centre, they are usually set up to make it easy to create a homely environment, where the lighting can be lowered, the room made comfortable and she can continue to relax as undisturbed as possible. In an obstetrics unit, it can be more difficult as it is likely to be set up differently. In this case, it would be down to you to see how you can make the lighting softer, maybe use the light in the en-suite bathroom rather than the main light in the room or ask for a lamp. Use a blanket from home and even her own pillow, something that reminds her of being cosy. She will probably have thought about this before going into labour, so ask her what she wants you to do when it comes to the room in which she will give birth, and then when the time comes, do it for her.

There can be times when medical staff such as midwives and doctors need to be in the room, but there are also times when they don't need to. It can be hard to relax fully when there are people in the room you don't know, especially if they are making noise. If this happens, you can ask them to either leave you both alone for a while to give Penelope the best chance of relaxing, or ask them to keep their voices at a low level if it is disturbing her. The next chapter explains how the environment not only impacts relaxation but also the hormones that she needs to produce to give birth.

WHAT TO DO WHEN THINGS GET TOUGH

There is a breathing technique that Penelope will be using to help her focus on something other than the contraction as it happens. Stare at your watch for a full minute. Or if you don't have a watch, use the timer on your phone or the clock on your computer. How long did that feel? I bet it felt like every second dragged. Now I want you to close your eyes and breathe in to the count of 5 and then out to the count of 5 six times. That was roughly the same amount of time but I can guarantee that the second time it felt like it went so much faster. This is why she will be breathing deeply during contractions. It not only helps with the relaxation, because it is pretty hard to breathe in and out slowly whilst tensing, but it also makes the whole thing seem to happen faster. As well as this, there is the fact that we place more importance on a feeling we are concentrating on. For example, did you notice how your tongue felt in your mouth until I just asked? My guess is that you hadn't even noticed it until I mentioned it and now it feels too big and all awkward, which is probably annoying you. If Penelope focuses completely on how the contraction feels, it becomes a much bigger sensation than if she is thinking about something else. That is not to say she won't feel it, but it will become easier for her to deal with. Before she goes into labour, she will have decided on some imagery that works with her breathing, so ask her what she has chosen. It could be the waves on the ocean, a balloon, the leaves on a tree. It could be anything at all, but knowing what she has selected will help you to get her back on track by asking her to visualise it. Whilst focussing on the imagery, she will be taking long, controlled breaths in and out.

There will be times when her oxytocin levels are higher than her endorphin levels and she might find it harder to do this. You might notice that she begins to tense her shoulders or that her jaws are locked together as she tries to breathe. First of all, ask her if she would like your help. She might not and this is fine, just do as much as you can to tell her what an amazing job she is doing. Depending on where she is, get in front of her if you can, ask her to focus on you and hold her hand. If she is at the stage where she needs to lean on a wall or you can't get in front of her, stand to the side of her and, if she doesn't mind, place your hands on her shoulders or waist. When the next contraction begins, ask her to copy your breathing. Take long slow breaths in and let them out as slowly as you can, trying to keep to a rhythm that she can manage. Stroke her jaw to help relax those muscles if they are tense, stroke her shoulders gently if you can, or down her back and arms. Anywhere that you can reach that seems tense.

As the labour progresses and the intensity of the contractions increases, Penelope will be looking for more ways to deal with them. She might want to lean on you, she might need you to rub the little dip in the small of her back to help with the pressure, she might choose to lean against a wall or use her birthing ball. She might also use a visualisation technique which can give her an extra level of comfort. It takes the idea of focusing on something other than the contraction one step further: she will take herself off into a daydream-like state in between contractions so that when one arrives it is much easier to cope with. The technique itself is extremely simple and one that you can help her with if she needs you to. She will find somewhere comfortable for her, close her eyes and imagine being stood at the top of a set of stone steps with her favourite place in nature at the bottom. With every breath out, she will relax her body and imagine going down each step, stopping to take a look around, until she has drifted off into a daydream.

For you, the main thing to do is to make sure she is in an environment that allows her to do this. Low lights and quiet are good, but if you are in the waiting room or the midwives have just arrived, it is not always possible, so make it work as best you can. The other way to help is to guide her with the imagery of the place in nature to get her there faster. If she is starting to struggle with the intensity of the contractions, offer to help her with this. Once she is comfy, ask her to imagine herself at the top of ten steps leading to her favourite place in nature. With each outbreath, count backwards from 10 down to 1. When at 1, ask her to look around and notice different things. Ask her what her favourite place looks like before labour begins so that you can point things out to her when helping her with this visualisation, for example maybe there is a lake, or mountains, or large oak trees etc. You can do soft-touch massage on her skin at the same time if it doesn't distract her. Once she is calmer and obviously more relaxed, stop talking and just be by her side in case she needs you again.

You can find examples of soft-touch massage and videos of birth partners using the techniques during labour at **www.keepcalmandbirthon.com** and you will need the password GXWYH.

WHAT TO DO IF LABOUR SLOWS DOWN

It can be really disheartening for a woman in labour if things suddenly stop or slow down. As the birth partner, there are things you can do to support her in staying positive and calm, as well as ways you can help to get things going again.

The first culprits are usually her hormones. They play a massive part during labour, so knowing how they work will give you the best chance of understanding why things speed up or slow down or sometimes even stop. I am going to concentrate on three hormones in this book, as knowing their effects will give you the best chance of understanding what is happening and why.

The first one is the big one: oxytocin. Oxytocin is what causes the uterus to contract. It is the hormone of love, and is produced when you feel loved, safe, and comfortable. When the baby is developed enough and is ready to be born, proteins are produced in his/her lungs which set off the chain reaction to tell Penelope's body it is time to begin producing oxytocin as well as all the other hormones it needs to do the job. Her body will carefully control the amount it produces to make sure that it never gives her more than she can handle. As the labour progresses and more oxytocin is released, the uterus tends to contracts harder and for longer, which is why birth gets more intense as it goes on.

The second hormone is endorphins. Endorphins are your body's natural pain relief. They are far stronger than any synthetic pain relief and interact with your brain to reduce your perception of pain, and they do exactly this during labour. You produce endorphins when you exercise and use your muscles more than normal, and they help to produce a sense of happiness and well-being, which is why exercise is always recommended to help those suffering from depression. During labour, Penelope's body will produce enough endorphins to deal with the strength of the contractions, and once she is coping better, then it will produce more oxytocin to increase the rate and strength of contractions, then increases the release of endorphins to counteract any pain caused by the muscle being used a lot.

Most people believe birth to go on a linear scale, that what they are experiencing at 4cm dilation is a world away from what they will experience at 9cm, because it must only get worse as the contractions increase in intensity. This misconception is often what causes a woman to give up on her ability to cope with labour and birth. Birth actually goes in waves. As the level of oxytocin increases, it is likely that she will feel like her labour has all of a sudden got difficult and hard to cope with, but after a short time the endorphin levels will rise so that she no longer experiences this level of pain or difficulty. After a while, the oxytocin will shoot up again, causing another stage of difficulty, but once again the endorphins will rise with it and take away those feelings. Eventually, there will come a stage where the oxytocin is causing the uterus to contract with such strength that it requires more concentration and movement for her to cope, but if she can spend early labour relaxing rather than tensing, it will mean she has far more energy to deal with these last contractions before the baby is born.

Then there is the third hormone: melatonin. Melatonin is most known for sleep. It is the hormone you release when you feel safe enough to let your guard down and sleep without any potential danger. It is why you often struggle to sleep in new places with new noises and new mattresses etc.: because the place is unfamiliar, until you are certain that there is no danger present, your body will not produce this hormone and won't allow you to rest properly. The production of melatonin in labour signals that the surroundings are safe enough to birth a vulnerable infant and that it is safe to continue to produce oxytocin to open the cervix.

Without the production of these three hormones, Penelope's body cannot birth the baby effectively, no matter how much she relaxes, so if things slow down, it is important to think about where you are and the environment you are in. If you are in a place full of bright lights, unfamiliar noises and new people, then it is likely her body will naturally stop producing the necessary hormones and the contractions will stop or become much less effective. Often women arrive at hospital and their hormones shut everything down. They then are told they need a drip to get things going again, which can lead to further intervention and they say how lucky they are that they were in hospital when it all happened otherwise the outcome could have been much worse, without realising that is was probably being in a hospital environment that caused it all in the first place. Her body won't care that the hospital is a safe place, it will care that her heart rate has elevated slightly and that she feels slightly nervous about the noises and that she doesn't know the person who is now trying to put their hand up her foof to see how far dilated she is. Had those other people known this, they could have asked for some privacy and created a space that made them feel loved, secure and safe enough that they could have gone to sleep there, and their bodies would have started producing the hormones again and everything would have carried on without the need for intervention. And this is something you need to remember. If there is no immediate danger to Penelope or the baby, then asking for privacy and recreating that perfect environment is the best and least intrusive way of getting everything going again.

The body has built-in mechanisms that are designed to keep everyone safe, and it won't give birth to that baby unless it decides it is okay to do so. Moving from home to the birth centre or hospital makes it think that you are moving because there is a danger present, because really women are built to stay where they are once labour is established, so until it feels settled in a new place that is safe, it won't start everything up again. Knowing this means that rather than giving up, you can take positive steps to get those important hormones going again. If there are other factors at play, such as Penelope or the baby being at risk, then there are other things to consider, and Chapter 4 will give you a formula to help you both make the right choices for the safety of Penelope and the baby.

If you are the dad or Penelope's partner, you can help the oxytocin to flow easily. As I said before, it is the hormone of love. It is produced when during an orgasm and is why the bump goes tight afterwards. Giving orgasms might not be high on your list of priorities whilst Penelope is in labour, but with this in mind it makes sense as to why being close, being by yourselves, cuddling and generally acting like loved-up teenagers will help to get those contractions going again. It doesn't have to even go as far as heavy petting to be effective; just lying next to each other, stroking each other's skin and feeling as though you are the only two people in the world is a surefire way to get the oxytocin pumping. If there is no risk to

Penelope or the baby, it is perfectly okay to ask everyone else to leave the room and be close together without the watchful eyes of the midwife putting you off. Believe it or not, in a lot of birth centres this kind of behaviour is actually encouraged by the midwives themselves, who know just how powerful feeling loved can be during labour.

If you are a friend, her parent or the adoptive parent of the baby, the above approach is obviously not appropriate. However, you can still help to create that feeling of love with hugs, stroking her arms, and generally making Penelope feel like she is surrounded by people who love her and make her feel safe. Keeping the environment calm and relaxing with people she knows and trusts will help massively as well. Laughter is another way of getting the oxytocin flowing, so telling jokes, watching funny videos together and recounting past adventures that make her laugh will be most helpful. It might take slightly longer but it will still work to get her body back on track. Laughter might seem counter-intuitive when creating a calm environment but the two together can be quite powerful.

If the endorphins are taking their time in helping her to cope with the sensations, then soft-touch massage can help stimulate them and increase their effectiveness, meaning you don't need to reach for the drugs just yet. To do this, gently and slowly run your fingertips and nails over the surface of the skin to create a tingly effect. It is more than worth practising during pregnancy to find out what and where works best for Penelope. Ask her where it feels the nicest, where it is the most effective and where it annoys her so you know exactly what to do when she needs you in labour (bearing in mind it may change then, though!). You can do it over the arms, shoulders, chest, back, legs, abdomen, through the hair and on the scalp. You can do it in between contractions if she is relaxing, or/and you can do it during a contraction if it helps, but make sure it is what she wants before you begin, as sometimes it can be distracting if she is trying to concentrate on her breathing.

WHAT TO DO IF CIRCUMSTANCES CHANGE

If Penelope has any special circumstances with her pregnancy, and she has read *Keep Calm and Birth On: 10 Ways to Survive Giving Birth*, she will already have looked into the different options available to her for her birth and have planned around those things. As a birth partner, it is important to be on board with her wishes so if there is anything that you don't understand or don't agree with, you need to talk to her about it. She needs full support in the birthing room, and not being fully on her side might mean her birth not going as she hopes. It is better to step down from the role than it is to pretend you fully accept her decisions. For most other women, the first time they come across the need to discuss what they want to happen is when they are told they need to be induced for going past their due date. This makes a lot of women truly believe that their body has failed them, which is not true as the reason most women haven't gone into labour yet is simply that the baby isn't ready. There are other pathways of care available and Penelope will be given the option of choosing these instead if she so wishes. If she does choose induction, it might be hard for Penelope to accept at such a late stage that all her plans for birth might need to change, so being there to support her is vital. She will still need a strong birth partner and the same environment around her as much as possible, and she will still want to use the same coping techniques, so your job in this case is to help her achieve as normal a birth as possible in the circumstances.

The same goes for if nature throws a spanner in the works and things do not go as smoothly as expected. If Penelope is being told she needs help with her labour, it can be hard to listen to what she is being told and deal with contractions at the same time. This is the time to step up as a birth partner, ask the right questions, get the answers and then feed them back to Penelope so she can make a choice as to what she would like to happen. If you are the dad or Penelope's partner, obviously this will need to be a joint decision for the health of both Penelope and the baby. Ultimately though, everything is Penelope's choice, it is *her* body, so it is important to listen to what she is saying and support her as best you can.

If you feel unsure about the choices being presented to you when you talk to the medical staff, there is a clever acronym you can use to remember what you need to know: BRAIN.

B – Benefits – what are the benefits of each option?

R – Risks – what are the risks of each option?

A – Alternatives – are there any alternatives we can discuss?

I – Instinct – what are your instincts telling you about how necessary the intervention is?

N – No – What are the risks if we refuse this treatment/option? What would be the next steps?

The main thing you need to remember is that everything to do with birth is a choice, and no one can tell you what you must do in any circumstances. Medical professionals can guide you both and give you their recommendations, but that does not mean that you have to do anything if it is not something you are okay with. For the vast majority of women, this is never an issue because they don't need special care and their birth goes smoothly, but for some women, knowing that they don't have to do something can empower them to have the best birth possible in the given circumstances, and Penelope will need your support with this if it becomes necessary. As her birth partner, you are her advocate as she may not be able to deal with her contractions and hold a proper conversation at the same time. If you find yourself in a situation where you have been told that Penelope has no option but to do as she is told, then you should first question why she is not being given a choice, and work through the BRAIN acronym. There are absolutely no restrictions when it comes to birth. It is not about going against medical advice just for the fun of it – Penelope wouldn't do that to herself or the baby – but sometimes it requires asking for an individual plan of care rather than the care providers just using a ready-made one. This is not your problem and Penelope is entitled to have her needs met, whatever the circumstances.

This is the biggest step in having a positive birth experience. Sometimes women's bodies and babies don't play ball. There is no one to blame, it is just unfortunate circumstances. However, Penelope might be feeling disappointed and confused about what happened and why, and it is important to get her to recognise that these feelings are okay and encourage her to talk to someone about them after the birth when she feels ready, if she doesn't do it for herself. Debriefs are available everywhere, where a midwife will take her, and you if you wish, through the birth and explain what happened. They are invaluable in helping both of you to understand how events unfolded and can fill in the gaps of why it had to be that way, rather than Penelope and you spending years wondering what went wrong.

Hopefully, all of this is going to be irrelevant to you anyway, as Penelope is going to have a straightforward, amazing birth, so the next chapter will tell you what to do when it is time for her to get that baby out.

WHAT TO DO WHEN BABY IS BORN

Once the cervix has moved out of the way of the baby's head, she is ready to move down the birth canal to be born. Now the contractions are working to slowly move her down towards the edge of the vagina so she can be pushed out into the big wide world. The key thing here is that there is no reason for Penelope to physically push the baby down and out, her body is capable of doing it all by itself. Yes, I am sorry, you don't actually get to shout 'PUUUUUSSSSHHHH!' like you see on the TV. Pushing is a self-perpetuating myth, where women expect to push because they believe they have to, so the midwives tell them when to push because the women are expecting it and will panic-push if they are not guided, and then because women are told to push, they believe they need to push to get the baby out. Crazy, really. When women feel this strange full sensation and the movement with each contraction, they sometimes think that this must be the urge to push and begin forcefully trying to push their baby down. This actually makes it more difficult for the baby to move through the birth canal because the act of pushing tenses up all the muscles, which prevents the baby from moving through as easily. So what Penelope can do to help is, instead of breathing out slowly as she would for the other contractions, to imagine the breath passing down through her body to help gently move the baby a little bit further down. She might even start humming. After a while, the baby will be far enough down the birth canal to be what we lovingly call 'ejected' into the world. At this point, she may feel a strong reaction or it may be slight, but her body will spasm a little, pushing the baby's head through the opening of the vagina. As it does this, it will open up the folded muscles within the vagina to allow the baby to move through with no or minimal tearing. In most cases, the baby's head will not move through the opening fully first time; in fact it can take a few goes before the vaginal muscles have opened up properly, so now Penelope just needs to relax as much as she can and let her body do its thing. This can be quite emotionally taxing because labour can be tiring and most women want it to be over at this point, so as a birth partner your job is to help Penelope to keep calm and encourage her to not give up, to let her body do what it needs to do, and to tell her what an amazing job she is doing. There are circumstances where tearing cannot be avoided, such as the baby having his/her hand by the side of his/her face, but in most cases this slow and calm process and everyone's patience will drastically reduce the chances of tearing. Once the baby's head has been born, usually the shoulders come with the next contraction, although in rare cases it can take one more. And *voilà!* That's it, baby is born and your work here is done. Well, almost.

There are positions Penelope can get into to help the baby move more easily. The best position is the one that uses gravity to move the baby down the birth canal and out, but wherever she is comfortable is more important. There is only one position that should be avoided when it comes to this final stage and that is lying on her back. This is the position seen in most films and TV programmes and is the one we assume is needed to give birth, but actually it makes the birthing bit extremely difficult. At the back of Penelope's pelvis is a small bone that acts like a trap door when the baby is moving through. If she lies on her back, the movement of this bone is restricted, making it harder for the baby because it reduces the space that s/he has to move down and kind of creates a hill for him/her to climb. The only reason this position has ever been used in birth is to give the doctor or the midwife a better view of what is going on, whereas a good doctor or midwife can do this regardless of the position the woman is in. Staying off the bed will make birth much easier but if Penelope can't, make sure she at least stays off her back.

Baby needs plenty of room to move through, so the second thing to remember is Penelope needs to keep her knees as wide apart as possible. Being upright is also preferable as it uses gravity to move the baby down faster, so encourage her to be on her knees or standing. As the birth partner, you may be needed to provide support for this, either by Penelope leaning on you or by holding her leg in the air if she is on the bed, or by holding her steady if she chooses to squat. She will instinctively know what to do; just allow her to move as and when she needs to, and make sure you help her to get into whichever position she wants to be in. Apart from that, there are really no other rules.

Once baby is out, Penelope will have skin-to-skin for as long as possible, and it is time to cut the cord. The cord is how the baby has been receiving the nutrients and oxygen s/he has needed from the placenta whilst s/he has been growing, so once the baby is born he no longer needs this cord and it will eventually fall off and leave a cute little belly button. Until recently in the UK, the cord used to be clamped almost immediately after the baby was born. This is still the case in many places around the world. However, roughly a third of the baby's blood is still in the placenta immediately after birth and, when left untouched, the cord carries on pulsating to move the blood from the placenta back into the baby, along with any stem cells left in the cord. Now, in the UK at least, the standard procedure is to allow the cord to pulsate for around 3 to 5 minutes after the baby is born, and then to clamp and cut the cord. There is also the option to 'wait for white', the term given for when mothers ask for the cord to be left alone until it has stopped pulsating completely and all the blood and stem cells are back into the baby. There is also such a thing as a 'lotus birth', where the cord isn't cut at all and the placenta is kept with the baby until the cord falls away all by itself. It is for Penelope to choose what she would like to happen with the cord once the baby is born, and for you to make sure it happens.

CONCLUSION

And that is pretty much what you need to know. Your job is important and plays a big part in keeping Penelope's birth the way she wants it to be. If you can remember the five key points below, then you will be the world's greatest birth partner:

- Create an environment around her that will allow her to relax and keep calm.
- Support her with her breathing and visualisation techniques if she is struggling with the intensity of the contractions at any point.
- If things slow down or stop, look around for any outside factors that may be affecting her hormones and fix them as much as possible. Do whatever is needed to get those hormones flowing again.
- Use the BRAIN acronym to make sure that her wishes are respected and upheld as much as possible.
- Support her in her chosen birthing position whilst encouraging her to keep breathing rather than forcefully pushing, and make sure

her request for what happens to the cord is honoured.

Simple.

I would like to thank you on behalf of your pregnant lady for taking the time to read this book. She will feel confident and supported during the birth, knowing that you have got her back and a great understanding of how to help her if she needs it. That in itself can make a massive difference in how well it goes.

Further reading :

Keep Calm and Birth On: 10 Ways to Survive Giving Birth is available at Amazon in kindle and paperback, and on Kobo as an eBook.

Printed in Great Britain
by Amazon

46312842R00031